Copyright © 2022 by Monica Dimitrios

All rights reserved. No part of this publication may be reproduced, distributed, or transmitted in any form or by any means, including photocopying, recording, or other electronic or mechanical methods, without the prior written permission of the publisher, except in the case of brief quotations embodied in critical reviews and certain other noncommercial uses permitted by copyright law.

Table of Contents

LONGEVITY DIET

The longevity diet recommends following a plant-based diet that includes little-to-no meat and poultry and periodic fasting. Although the diet was designed for older adults, it has potential health payoffs for people of every age and stage of life.

LONGEVITY DIET RECIPES

1. Italian-Herbed Chicken and Mozzarella Melts

Prep Time: 20 mins

Total Time: 3 hrs 35 mins

Servings: 8

Ingredients

- 8 skinless, boneless chicken thighs (about 2 pounds total)
- 2 medium green sweet peppers, thinly sliced
- ½ teaspoon dried rosemary, crushed
- 1 cup bottled spaghetti sauce
- ½ cup coarsely chopped pitted Kalamata olives
- 1 cup shredded part-skim mozzarella cheese (4 ounces)
- ¼ cup snipped fresh basil
- 2 tablespoons grated Parmesan cheese
- 8 slices whole grain Italian bread
- 8 slices Apple slices

Directions

1. Lightly coat a 3 1/2- or 4-quart slow cooker with cooking spray. Lightly coat a large nonstick skillet with cooking spray. Heat the skillet over medium-high heat. Add chicken; cook about 2 minutes or until light brown on both sides, turning once.

2. Place sweet peppers in prepared slow cooker. Top with chicken. Sprinkle with rosemary. Pour spaghetti sauce over chicken.

3. Cover and cook on low-heat setting for 6 1/2 to 7 hours or on high-heat setting for 3 1/4 to 3 1/2 hours.

4. Preheat broiler. Line a baking sheet with foil; set aside. Using a slotted spoon transfer peppers and chicken to a medium bowl, reserving cooking juices. Using two forks pull chicken apart into coarse shreds. Add olives to chicken. In a small bowl combine mozzarella cheese, basil, and Parmesan cheese.

5. Place bread on prepared baking sheet. Broil 4 to 5 inches from the heat for 1 to 2 minutes or until toasted. Turn over bread slices. Top each slice

with some of the chicken mixture; drizzle each with about 1 tablespoon of the cooking juices. Sprinkle each with cheese mixture. Broil 1 to 2 minutes more or until toasted and cheese is melted. If desired, serve with apple.

Total Time: 45 mins

Servings: 6

Ingredients

- 1 tablespoon extra-virgin olive oil
- 2 tablespoons all-purpose flour
- 2 ½ cups low-fat milk, heated
- 1/2 cup grated fontina cheese, divided
- ½ teaspoon ground nutmeg
- Salt & freshly ground pepper, to taste
- 1 pound fresh or frozen cheese tortellini, preferably low-fat
- ¼ cup fine dry breadcrumbs
- 2 tablespoons freshly grated Parmesan cheese

Directions

1. Preheat oven to 350 degrees F. Coat 6 individual gratin dishes or a 1 1/2-quart shallow baking dish with cooking spray. Put a large pot of water on to boil for cooking pasta.

2. Heat oil in a large saucepan over medium heat. Add flour and cook, whisking constantly, for 1 to 2 minutes. Add hot milk and bring to a simmer, whisking, until smooth and slightly thickened, 3 to 4 minutes. Remove from heat and add 1/4 cup fontina and nutmeg, stirring to melt the cheese. Season with salt and pepper.

3. Meanwhile, cook tortellini until just tender, 6 to 8 minutes or according to package directions. Drain and rinse well.

4. Combine the tortellini with the cheese sauce and toss. Transfer to the prepared dishes or baking dish. Top with the remaining 1/4 cup fontina. Combine breadcrumbs and Parmesan and sprinkle evenly over the tortellini.

5. Bake the tortellini until golden and bubbly, 15 to 25 minutes. Serve immediately.

3. Lasagna di Pesce Seafood Lasagna

Prep Time: 45 mins

Total Time: 1 hr 30 mins

Servings: 8

Ingredients

- 8 ounces no-boil lasagna noodles
- 2 cups bottled clam juice
- 1 cup white wine
- 1 cup water
- 1 pound fresh medium shrimp, peeled, deveined and chopped
- 1 pound fresh Pacific sole fillet, cut into 1/2-inch pieces
- 8 ounces fresh salmon fillet, skinned and cut into 1/2-inch pieces
- 2 ½ tablespoons extra-virgin olive oil, divided
- 2 tablespoons finely chopped shallot
- 3 anchovy fillets, rinsed and chopped
- 2 cloves garlic, minced
- 12 ounces fresh mushrooms, sliced (4 cups)

- ⅓ cup chopped fresh basil
- Salt & freshly ground pepper, to taste
- ⅓ cup all-purpose flour
- 2 tablespoons lemon juice
- Pinch of cayenne
- ⅓ cup fine dry breadcrumbs
- 2 tablespoons freshly grated Parmesan cheese
- 2 tablespoons chopped fresh parsley

Directions

1. Place lasagna noodles in a large bowl of warm water and let soak, stirring occasionally, until pliable, at least 10 minutes.

2. Meanwhile, combine clam juice, wine and water in a large deep skillet. Bring to a simmer. Reduce heat to medium-low and add shrimp. Poach until pink, about 40 seconds. Remove with a slotted spoon and transfer to a colander over a bowl.

3. Add sole and salmon to poaching liquid. Poach until just opaque, about 1 minute. Remove with a slotted spoon and place in colander with shrimp.

Let drain. Strain poaching liquid through a fine sieve and set aside. Wipe pan dry.

4. Heat 1 1/2 teaspoons oil in the pan over medium-high heat. Add shallots, anchovies and garlic and cook, mashing anchovies into a paste, for about 1 minute. Add mushrooms and saute until browned, about 2 minutes. Add basil and season with salt and pepper. Transfer to colander with the seafood. Add any accumulated juices to the reserved poaching liquid. Measure out 3 1/2 cups hot liquid, adding water if necessary.

5. Heat the remaining 2 tablespoons oil in a large heavy saucepan over medium heat. Add flour and cook, whisking constantly, for 1 minute. Add the reserved poaching liquid and bring to a simmer, whisking, until smooth and thickened to the consistency of heavy cream, 5 to 6 minutes. Add lemon juice and season with salt, pepper and cayenne. Reserve 1 1/2 cups sauce; gently mix seafood mixture into remaining sauce.

6. Preheat oven to 350 degrees F. Coat a 9-by-13-1/2-inch baking dish with cooking spray.

7. Spoon 1/2 cup reserved sauce into the prepared dish. Drain the noodles and blot dry. Alternate 4 layers of noodles and 3 layers of the seafood mixture in dish, starting and ending with noodles. Spread remaining 1 cup sauce over the top, coating the noodles completely.

8. Cover the lasagna with foil and bake for 25 minutes. Uncover, sprinkle with breadcrumbs and Parmesan and bake until golden and bubbly, 15 to 20 minutes more. Let stand for 10 minutes. Garnish with parsley and serve.

Total Time: 35 mins

Servings: 4

Ingredients

- 4 teaspoons extra-virgin olive oil, divided
- 1 16-ounce tube prepared plain polenta, cut into 1/2-inch cubes
- 1 clove garlic,minced
- 1 small onion, halved and thinly sliced
- 1 red bell pepper, diced
- 1/2 teaspoon paprika, preferably smoked, plus more for garnish
- 1 15-ounce can butter beans, rinsed
- 4 cups packed baby spinach
- ¾ cup vegetable broth
- ½ cup shredded Manchego or Monterey Jack cheese
- 2 teaspoons sherry vinegar

Directions

1. Heat 2 teaspoons oil in a large nonstick skillet over medium-high heat. Add polenta and cook in a single layer, stirring occasionally, until beginning to brown, 8 to 10 minutes. Transfer to a plate.

2. Reduce the heat to medium, add the remaining 2 teaspoons oil and garlic to the pan, and cook, stirring, until fragrant, 30 seconds. Add onion and bell pepper; cook, stirring, until just tender, 3 to 5 minutes. Sprinkle with paprika; cook, stirring, for 30 seconds. Stir in beans, spinach and broth; cook, stirring, until the beans are heated through and the spinach is wilted, 2 to 3 minutes. Remove from the heat; stir in cheese and vinegar. Serve vegetables over polenta. Sprinkle with paprika, if desired.

5. Quick Lentil Salmon Salad

Total Time: 30 mins

Servings: 4

Ingredients

- ¾ cup brown lentils
- ½ cup chopped red onion plus 1/4 cup thinly sliced, divided
- 2 cloves garlic, minced
- ¾ teaspoon salt
- ¼ cup extra-virgin olive oil
- 3 tablespoons red-wine vinegar
- ¾ teaspoon dried thyme
- ¼ teaspoon ground pepper
- 1 15-ounce can salmon, drained
- 1 cup carrot ribbons
- 1 cup sliced celery
- 4 lemon wedges for serving

Directions

1. Bring a medium saucepan of water to a boil. Add lentils and chopped onion, reduce heat to maintain a lively simmer and cook until the lentils are just tender, 11 to 13 minutes. Drain well.

2. Meanwhile, mash garlic and salt into a paste with the side of a chef's knife (or a fork). Transfer to a medium bowl and whisk in oil, vinegar, thyme and pepper.

3. Remove any skin and/or bones from salmon; flake the salmon into a large bowl. Add sliced onion, carrot and 3 tablespoons of the dressing; gently toss to coat. Add celery and the lentils to the remaining dressing; gently stir to combine. Divide the lentils among 4 bowls, top with the salmon salad and serve with lemon wedges.

6. Corn & Broccoli Calzones

Total Time: 45 mins

Servings: 6

Ingredients

- 1 ½ cups chopped broccoli florets
- 1 1/2 cups fresh corn kernels
- 1 cup shredded part-skim mozzarella cheese
- ⅔ cup part-skim ricotta cheese
- 4 scallions, thinly sliced
- ¼ cup chopped fresh basil
- ½ teaspoon garlic powder
- ¼ teaspoon salt
- ¼ teaspoon freshly ground pepper

Directions

1. Position racks in upper and lower thirds of oven; preheat to 475 degrees F. Coat 2 baking sheets with cooking spray.
2. Combine broccoli, corn, mozzarella, ricotta, scallions, basil, garlic powder, salt and pepper in a large bowl.

3. On a lightly floured surface, divide dough into 6 pieces. Roll each piece into an 8-inch circle. Place a generous 3/4 cup filling on one half of each circle, leaving a 1-inch border of dough. Brush the border with water and fold the top half over the filling. Fold the edges over and crimp with a fork to seal. Make several small slits in the top to vent steam; brush each calzone with oil. Transfer the calzones to the prepared baking sheets.

4. Bake the calzones, switching the pans halfway through, until browned on top, about 15 minutes. Let cool slightly before serving.

Total Time: 15 mins

Servings: 4

Ingredients

- 4 thick slices whole-wheat bread
- 6 tablespoons light brown sugar
- 1 teaspoon grated lemon zest
- 2 teaspoons lemon juice
- 3 cups sliced or diced hulled strawberries
- 4 tablespoons mascarpone

Directions

1. Toast bread in a toaster.
2. Meanwhile, heat a large skillet over high heat. Add sugar, lemon zest and lemon juice and cook, stirring, until the sugar melts and the mixture begins to bubble, 30 seconds to 1 minute. Add strawberries and stir until juices begin to exude and the berries are heated through, 30 seconds to 1 minute more.

3. Spread 1 tablespoon mascarpone on each piece of toast. Top with the warm berries.

Total Time: 50 mins

Servings: 8

Ingredients

- 4 large lemons, divided, plus more for garnish
- 8 large artichokes
- 2 cups water
- 6 cloves garlic, chopped
- ¼ cup chopped fresh dill, plus more for garnish
- 1 teaspoon salt
- ¼ teaspoon ground pepper
- 1 ½ tablespoons extra-virgin olive oil

Directions

1. Squeeze the juice from 2 lemons. Fill a large bowl of cold water and add the juice and rinds. Use a paring knife to trim the bottom 1/4 inch off the artichoke stems. Snip the thorn off the leaves with kitchen shears. Cut off about 1 inch from the tops. With a melon baller or spoon, scoop out the fuzzy

chokes. Place the trimmed artichokes in the lemon water to prevent discoloration.

2. Squeeze 1/3 cup juice from the remaining 2 lemons. Combine the juice with 2 cups water in a large nonreactive pot wide enough to hold the artichokes in a single layer. Drain the artichokes and lay them on their sides in the pot. Top with garlic, dill, salt and pepper. Bring to a boil. Reduce heat to low, cover and simmer, turning the artichokes once, until tender when pierced with a fork, 18 to 20 minutes.

3. With a slotted spoon, transfer the artichokes to a deep platter. Simmer the liquid remaining in the pan over medium-high heat until reduced to 1 1/4 cups, about 10 minutes; spoon over the artichokes. Let cool to room temperature.

4. To serve, drizzle the artichokes with oil and baste with sauce. Garnish with chopped dill and lemon wedges, if desired.

9. Mediterranean Edamame Toss

Prep Time: 20 mins

Total Time: 35 mins

Servings: 4

Ingredients

- ½ cup uncooked quinoa, rinsed and drained
- 1 cup water
- 1 cup ready-to-eat fresh or frozen, thawed shelled sweet soybeans (edamame)
- 2 medium tomatoes, seeded and chopped
- 1 cup fresh arugula or spinach leaves
- ½ cup chopped red onion
- 2 tablespoons olive oil
- 1 teaspoon finely shredded lemon peel
- 2 tablespoons lemon juice
- ¼ cup crumbled reduced-fat feta cheese
- 2 tablespoons snipped fresh basil
- ¼ teaspoon salt
- ¼ teaspoon freshly ground black pepper

Directions

1. In a medium saucepan, combine quinoa and water. Bring to boiling; reduce heat. Cover and simmer about 15 minutes or until quinoa is tender and liquid is absorbed, adding edamame the last 4 minutes of cooking.
2. In a large bowl, combine quinoa mixture, tomato, arugula, and onion.
3. In a small bowl, whisk together olive oil, lemon peel, and lemon juice. Stir in half of the cheese, the basil, salt, and pepper. Add mixture to quinoa mixture, tossing to coat. Sprinkle with remaining half of the cheese. Serve at room temperature.

10. Very Versatile Roasted Red Pepper Sauce

Prep Time: 45 mins

Total Time: 1 hr

Servings: 12

Ingredients

- 1 ½ pounds red bell peppers (3-4 medium)
- 3 large cloves garlic, unpeeled
- 2 teaspoons smoked paprika
- 1 teaspoon kosher salt
- ¼ teaspoon cayenne pepper
- 1 ½ tablespoons balsamic vinegar, preferably aged
- 3 tablespoons extra-virgin olive oil

Directions

1. Position a rack in upper third of oven; preheat broiler. Line a baking sheet with foil.
2. Halve peppers lengthwise and discard stems and seeds. Place the halves, cut-side down, on the prepared pan along with garlic.

3. Broil, flipping often, until the peppers are charred in many spots, 10 to 15 minutes. Transfer the peppers to a bowl and loosely cover with the foil. Let stand until cool enough to handle, about 20 minutes. Place the garlic on a small plate.

4. Peel the peppers and garlic. Transfer the garlic to a food processor and add paprika, salt and cayenne; process to finely chop the garlic. Add the peppers and vinegar; process until pureed. With the machine running, slowly pour in oil through the feed tube. Let the sauce stand for 10 minutes before serving.

11. Quinoa Salad with Seared Tuna

Prep Time: 30 mins

Total Time: 50 mins

Servings: 6

Ingredients

- 12 ounces fresh or frozen tuna steaks
- 1 ½ cups quinoa
- 3 cups water
- ¼ teaspoon salt
- 1 large tomato, chopped
- 1 cup cucumber, seeded and chopped
- ½ cup crumbled reduced-fat feta cheese
- ¼ cup chopped red onion
- 2 tablespoons olive oil
- 2 tablespoons lemon juice
- 1 teaspoon honey
- ½ teaspoon snipped fresh oregano or 1/4 teaspoon dried oregano, crushed
- ¼ teaspoon ground black pepper
- Nonstick cooking spray

- ⅛ teaspoon salt
- ⅛ teaspoon ground black pepper

Directions

1. Thaw tuna steaks, if frozen. Rinse quinoa well in a fine mesh sieve. Bring water and 1/4 teaspoon salt to boiling. Add quinoa; reduce heat. Cover and simmer 15 minutes or until most of the water is absorbed and quinoa is tender. Drain, if necessary. Spread on a baking sheet to cool slightly.
2. On a serving platter, combine quinoa, tomato, cucumber, feta cheese and red onion.
3. In a screw-top jar, combine olive oil, lemon juice, honey, 1/2 teaspoon oregano and pepper. Cover and shake well to combine. Add to quinoa mixture and toss to combine.
4. Lightly coat a grill pan or large skillet with nonstick cooking spray. Sprinkle tuna steaks with 1/8 teaspoon salt and the pepper. Cook on grill pan over medium-high heat 4 to 6 minutes per 1/2-inch thickness of fish, turning once or until browned on both sides and fish begins to flake

when tested with a fork and center is just pink.
Thinly slice tuna steaks and serve atop salad.
Garnish with fresh oregano.

12. Pan-Fried Zucchini Chips

Prep Time: 40 mins

Total Time: 40 mins

Servings: 8

Ingredients

- ⅓ cup all-purpose flour
- 3 eggs, beaten
- 1 cup whole-wheat panko or breadcrumbs
- ⅓ cup grated Parmesan cheese
- Zest of 1 lemon
- 2 medium zucchini, cut into 1/4-inch-thick slices
- ½ cup avocado oil, divided
- ½ teaspoon coarse kosher salt

Directions

1. Preheat oven to 175 degrees F. Place a wire rack inside a large rimmed baking sheet.
2. Place flour and eggs in separate shallow bowls. Combine panko (or breadcrumbs), Parmesan and lemon zest in a third shallow bowl. Dredge

zucchini slices in the flour, shaking off any excess. Next, dip the zucchini in the eggs, turning to coat. Then, dredge in the breadcrumb mixture.

3. Heat 1/4 cup oil in a large nonstick skillet over medium-high heat. Reduce heat to medium and add about one-fourth of the zucchini rounds. Cook, turning once, until browned and crispy, 1 to 2 minutes total. Transfer to the prepared rack and baking sheet and place in the oven to keep warm. Repeat with the remaining zucchini, adding the remaining 1/4 cup oil halfway through. Sprinkle with salt and serve immediately.

13. Roasted Barramundi with Asparagus Gremolata

Prep Time: 25 mins

Total Time: 25 mins

Servings: 4

Ingredients

- 1 pound asparagus, trimmed
- 4 tablespoons extra-virgin olive oil, divided
- ½ teaspoon salt, divided
- ½ teaspoon ground pepper, divided
- 1 pound barramundi or mahi-mahi, skinned and cut into 4 portions
- 2 tablespoons lemon zest
- 4 tablespoons lemon juice, divided
- ½ cup chopped fresh parsley
- 1 large clove garlic, grated

Directions

1. Preheat oven to 450 degrees F. Coat a baking sheet with cooking spray.

2. Thinly slice 1/2 cup asparagus and set aside. Toss the remaining asparagus in a large bowl with 1 tablespoon oil and 1/4 teaspoon each salt and pepper. Spread on the prepared baking sheet. Place fish on top of the asparagus. Drizzle the fish with 2 tablespoons lemon juice and 1 tablespoon oil and season with the remaining 1/4 teaspoon each salt and pepper. Roast until the fish flakes easily with a fork, 6 to 10 minutes.

3. Meanwhile, combine the reserved asparagus with lemon zest, parsley, garlic and the remaining 2 tablespoons oil and 2 tablespoons lemon juice in the bowl. Serve the gremolata on top of the fish.

14. Salmon and Couscous Casserole

Prep Time: 15 mins

Total Time: 25 mins

Servings: 4

Ingredients

- 1 cup water
- 2 cloves garlic, minced
- ⅔ cup whole wheat couscous
- 1 (14.75 ounce) can salmon, drained, flaked, and skin and bones removed
- 2 cups packaged fresh baby spinach leaves
- ½ cup jarred roasted red sweet peppers, drained and chopped
- ⅓ cup jarred tomato bruschetta topper
- 2 tablespoons purchased toasted almonds

Directions

1. In a 2-quart microwave-safe casserole, combine the water and garlic. Microwave, uncovered, on 100% power (high) for 2-1/2 to 3 minutes or until

mixture is boiling. Remove from microwave and stir in couscous; spoon salmon atop couscous mixture. Cover and let stand for 5 minutes.

2. Add spinach, roasted peppers, and bruschetta topper to couscous mixture. Toss to combine. Divide mixture among four serving plates. Top with almonds. Makes 4 servings (1-1/4 cups each).

15. Rosemary-Goat Cheese Toast

Total Time: 5 mins

Servings: 1

Ingredients

- 1 diagonal slice baguette (1/4 inch thick), preferably whole-wheat
- 1 ½ tablespoons goat cheese
- ¼ teaspoon chopped fresh rosemary
- 1 teaspoon honey

Directions

1. Toast bread. Top with goat cheese and rosemary. Drizzle with honey.

16. Spaghetti alla Carbonara

Total Time: 40 mins

Servings: 6

Ingredients

- 1 teaspoon extra-virgin olive oil
- 3 ounces thinly sliced prosciutto, or Canadian bacon, trimmed of fat and diced (1/2 cup)
- 2 cloves garlic, minced
- Pinch of crushed red pepper
- 3 large eggs, (pasteurized, if desired)
- ¾ cup reduced-sodium chicken broth
- ¾ teaspoon freshly ground pepper
- 12 ounces whole-wheat spaghetti, or linguine
- 8 ounces broccolini, (2 1/2 cups) or broccoli rabe (4 cups), stem ends trimmed, cut into 1/2-inch pieces
- ⅓ cup freshly grated Parmesan or Pecorino Romano cheese
- Salt, to taste

Directions

1. Put a large pot of water on to boil for cooking pasta. Also bring about 1 inch of water to a gentle simmer in the bottom of a double boiler.

2. Heat oil in a medium nonstick skillet over medium heat. Add prosciutto (or Canadian bacon) and cook, stirring often, until heated through, about 2 minutes. Add garlic and crushed red pepper; cook, stirring, for 30 seconds. Remove from heat.

3. Whisk eggs, broth and pepper in the top of the double boiler to combine. Set over the simmering water in the bottom of the double boiler and cook, whisking constantly in a slow, steady, figure-eight motion, until the sauce steams and thickens enough to coat a metal spoon, 5 to 7 minutes. The sauce may have a few small curdles. Remove the top pan from the heat and whisk the sauce rapidly so it does not continue to curdle.

4. Meanwhile, cook pasta in the boiling water, stirring often, for 5 minutes. Drop in broccolini (or broccoli rabe) and cook until the pasta is

tender but firm, 4 to 6 minutes more. Drain and place in a large bowl. Add the egg sauce, the prosciutto (or bacon) mixture and cheese; toss to coat well. Season with salt, if desired.

17. Escarole & White Bean Salad with Swordfish

Total Time: 30 mins

Servings: 4

Ingredients

- ¼ cup extra-virgin olive oil
- 2 tablespoons lemon juice
- 1 teaspoon Dijon mustard
- ½ teaspoon salt, divided
- ½ teaspoon ground pepper, divided
- 1 15-ounce can white beans, rinsed
- 2 10-ounce swordfish steaks
- 1 teaspoon herbes de Provence
- 12 cups chopped escarole
- ¼ cup very thinly sliced red onion

Directions

1. Position rack in upper third of oven; preheat broiler to high. Line a broiler-safe pan with foil.
2. Whisk oil, lemon juice, mustard and 1/4 teaspoon each salt and pepper in a large bowl. Transfer 2 tablespoons of the dressing to a small bowl. Add

beans to the dressing in the large bowl and toss to combine.

3. Cut each swordfish steak in half so you have 4 equal portions; sprinkle with herbes de Provence and the remaining 1/4 teaspoon each salt and pepper. Place the fish on the prepared pan and broil on the upper rack until it just barely flakes when pressed with a knife, 8 to 10 minutes.

4. Toss escarole and onion with the beans. Serve the salad with the swordfish, drizzled with the reserved 2 tablespoons dressing.

Total Time: 20 mins

Servings: 4

Ingredients

- 1 small red onion, thinly sliced
- ¼ cup balsamic vinegar
- 4 10-inch whole-wheat tortillas
- 1 cup shredded sharp Cheddar cheese
- 8 slices deli turkey, preferably smoked (8 ounces)

Directions

1. Combine onion and vinegar in a bowl; let marinate for 5 minutes. Drain, reserving the vinegar for another use, such as salad dressing.

2. Warm 2 tortillas in a large nonstick skillet over medium-high heat for about 45 seconds, then flip. Pull the tortillas up the edges of the pan so they are no longer overlapping. Working on one half of each tortilla, sprinkle one-fourth of the cheese, cover with 2 slices of turkey and top with one-fourth of the onion. Fold the tortillas in half,

flatten gently with a spatula and cook until the cheese starts to melt, about 2 minutes. Flip and cook until the second side is golden, 1 to 2 minutes more.

3. Transfer to a plate and cover to keep warm. Make 2 more quesadillas with the remaining ingredients.

19. Baked Mushroom Rice

Total Time: 1 hr 20 mins

Servings: 4

Ingredients

- 1 ounce dried porcini mushrooms, (1 1/2 cups)
- 1 ½ cups hot water
- 4 teaspoons extra-virgin olive oil, divided
- 1 medium leek, trimmed, washed and sliced (1 cup)
- 1 cup short-grain brown rice, (see Ingredient notes)
- 2 cloves garlic, minced
- 1 tablespoon chopped fresh thyme, or 1 teaspoon dried
- ½ cup dry white wine
- 3 cups reduced-sodium chicken broth
- 4 ounces cremini, or baby bella mushrooms, wiped clean, stemmed and quartered
- ½ cup freshly grated Parmesan cheese
- ¼ cup chopped fresh parsley, divided
- 2 teaspoons balsamic vinegar

- ¼ teaspoon salt, or to taste

Directions

1. Combine porcini and hot water in a small bowl. Let stand for 30 minutes. Strain, reserving the liquid. Rinse the mushrooms well under cool water; drain and chop finely. Strain the reserved liquid through a coffee filter or paper towel to remove any sand or dirt.

2. Preheat oven to 425 degrees F.

3. Heat 2 teaspoons oil in a Dutch oven or large ovenproof high-sided skillet over medium heat. Add leek and the porcini; cook, stirring often, until the leek is tender, 2 to 3 minutes. Add rice, garlic and thyme; stir to coat well. Add wine and cook until almost all evaporated, 2 to 4 minutes. Add broth and the reserved porcini liquid. Bring to a boil. Cover the pan and transfer to the oven.

4. Bake until the rice is just tender but still has a little resistance and a creamy consistency, 40 to 50 minutes. If the risotto seems soupy, place it on the stovetop over medium heat and simmer for a

few minutes, stirring, until it reaches the desired consistency.

5. While the risotto is baking, heat the remaining 2 teaspoons oil in a nonstick skillet over medium-high heat. Add cremini and cook, stirring occasionally, until tender and browned, 5 to 7 minutes.

6. When the risotto is ready, stir in the cremini, Parmesan, 2 tablespoons parsley, vinegar, salt and pepper. Sprinkle the remaining parsley on top and serve immediately.

20. Baked Risotto Primavera

Total Time: 1 hr 10 mins

Servings: 6

Ingredients

- 1 tablespoon extra-virgin olive oil
- 2 medium onions, chopped (about 1 1/2 cups)
- 1 cup short- or medium-grain brown rice, (see Ingredient note)
- 3 cloves garlic, minced
- ½ cup dry white wine
- 2 14-1/2-ounce can reduced-sodium chicken broth, or 3 1/2 cups vegetable broth
- 8 ounces asparagus, ends trimmed, cut into 1-inch pieces (2 cups)
- 1 cup sugar snap peas, or snow peas, trimmed, cut into 1-inch pieces
- 1 cup diced red bell pepper, (1 medium)
- 1 1/2 cups freshly grated Parmesan cheese, (3 1/2 ounces)
- ¼ cup chopped fresh parsley
- ¼ cup chopped fresh chives

- 1-2 teaspoons freshly grated lemon zest

Directions

1. Preheat oven to 425 degrees F.
2. Heat oil in a Dutch oven or ovenproof high sided skillet over medium heat. Add onions and cook, stirring occasionally, until softened, 3 to 5 minutes. Stir in rice and garlic; cook, stirring, 1 to 2 minutes. Stir in wine and simmer until it has mostly evaporated. Add broth and bring to a boil. Cover the pan and transfer to the oven.
3. Bake until the rice is just tender, 50 minutes to 1 hour.
4. Shortly before the risotto is done, steam asparagus, peas and bell pepper until crisp-tender, about 4 minutes.
5. Fold the steamed vegetables, Parmesan, parsley, chives, lemon zest and pepper into the risotto. Serve immediately.

21. Sun-Dried Tomato Gnocchi

Total Time: 2 hrs 15 mins

Servings: 6

Ingredients

- 2 pounds medium Yukon Gold or russet potatoes
- ¾ teaspoon salt
- 1 large egg yolk, beaten
- 1/3 cup sun-dried tomatoes (not oil-packed)
- 1/4 cups all-purpose flour, divided

Directions

1 Preheat oven to 400 degrees F.

2 Pierce potatoes in several spots with a fork. Bake directly on the center rack until tender when pierced with a knife, 45 minutes to 1 1/4 hours, depending on the size and type of your potatoes. Remove to a wire rack and let stand until cool enough to handle, 15 to 20 minutes.

3 Scoop the insides out of the potato skins and push through a potato ricer fitted with a fine disc onto a clean counter. (If you don't have a ricer, mash the

potatoes until smooth.) Gather the potato into a mound on the counter, sprinkle with salt and let cool, about 15 minutes.

4   Meanwhile, soak sun-dried tomatoes in boiling water until soft, 10 to 20 minutes. Place the egg yolk in a food processor. Drain the tomatoes; transfer to the food processor with the yolk; pulse until pureed.

5   Put a large pot of water on to boil.

6   Pour tomato puree over the cooled potato and then sprinkle 1 cup flour on top. Use a bench knife or metal spatula to gently fold the flour and tomato puree into the potatoes until combined (it will not look like dough at this point). Gently squeeze, knead and pat the dough until it holds together and resembles biscuit dough or cookie dough. The dough will be a little sticky; if it's very sticky, add more flour, about 1 tablespoon at a time, as necessary. Be careful not to overwork the dough: overworked dough will yield tougher gnocchi.

7   Pat the dough into a 1 1/2-inch-thick disk and then divide it into 4 equal pieces. Working on a lightly floured surface with lightly floured hands, roll each portion into a 24- to 26-inch-long "snake," 1/2 to 3/4

inch wide. Start at the center of the dough and roll out using your fingertips and very light pressure; gently pull the dough out as you roll. Cut the snake into 3/4-inch pieces. Use your fingertip to make an indentation (or "dimple") in the center of each gnocchi. Place the gnocchi on a lightly floured baking sheet as they are made. Repeat with remaining dough.

8   Adjust the heat so the water is at a gentle boil. Add about one-quarter of the gnocchi at a time. When the gnocchi float to the top, transfer to a parchment or wax paper-lined baking sheet with a slotted spoon. Continue boiling the gnocchi in batches until they are all cooked, returning the water to a gentle boil between batches. Serve immediately or see Sauteed Gnocchi.

22. Herb-Crusted Mediterranean Sea Bass

Prep Time: 25 mins

Total Time: 1 hr 25 mins

Servings: 6

Ingredients

- 1 (3 pound) whole black bass or sea bass, cleaned, head and tail intact
- 2 tablespoons chopped fresh tarragon
- ¾ teaspoon salt, divided
- 3 tablespoons extra-virgin olive oil, divided
- ⅓ cup dry white wine
- 1 tablespoon butter
- 2 cloves garlic, minced
- 1 ½ cups whole-wheat breadcrumbs
- 3 tablespoons chopped fresh basil
- 3 tablespoons chopped fresh marjoram or oregano
- 3 tablespoons chopped fresh parsley

Directions

1   Preheat oven to 350 degrees F.

2   Sprinkle the inside of the fish cavity with tarragon and 1/4 teaspoon salt.

3   Heat 2 tablespoons oil in a roasting pan over medium-low heat. Add the fish and pour in wine. Bake until the fish is opaque in the center, 40 to 50 minutes.

4   Meanwhile, heat the remaining 1 tablespoon oil, butter and garlic in a large skillet over medium heat. Add breadcrumbs, basil, marjoram (or oregano), parsley and the remaining 1/2 teaspoon salt. Cook, stirring often, until the breadcrumbs are toasted, 3 to 4 minutes.

5   Score the skin of the fish near the gills and carefully pull it off toward the tail. (Discard the skin.) Spread the breadcrumb mixture over the fish, pressing gently. Return the fish to the oven and bake for 5 minutes.

Total Time: 10 mins

Servings: 16

Ingredients

- 16 thin slices prosciutto
- 16 whole pitted dates

Directions

1   Wrap a slice of prosciutto around each date. Grind pepper on top.

24. Lovage Pesto

Prep Time: 10 mins

Total Time: 10 mins

Servings: 20

Ingredients

- 1 stalk green garlic or 2 large cloves garlic
- ½ cup Marcona almonds
- cups loosely packed fresh lovage
- 1 cup extra-virgin olive oil , divided
- ¼ cup fresh basil
- ¼ cup grated Parmesan or pecorino cheese
- ½ teaspoon lemon zest
- tablespoons lemon juice
- 1 teaspoon salt
- ½ teaspoon ground pepper

Directions

1. Combine garlic and almonds in a food processor. Pulse until coarsely chopped, scraping down the

sides once. Add lovage, 1/2 cup oil, basil and cheese. Process until coarsely chopped. Add lemon zest, lemon juice, salt, pepper and the remaining 1/2 cup oil. Process, scraping down the sides once

25. Roasted Florets

Total Time: 30 mins

Servings: 4

Ingredients

- cups bite-size cauliflower florets, or broccoli florets (about 1 head), sliced
- tablespoons extra-virgin olive oil
- ½ teaspoon salt, or to taste
- Freshly ground pepper, to taste

Directions

1. Preheat oven to 450 degrees F. Place florets in a large bowl with oil, salt and pepper and toss to coat. Spread out on a baking sheet. Roast the vegetables, stirring once, until tender-crisp and browned in spots, 15 to 25 minutes. Serve hot or warm with lemon wedges, if desired.

Total Time: 1 hr

Servings: 4

Ingredients

- tablespoons extra-virgin olive oil, divided
- 1 large red onion, halved and thinly sliced
- ½ teaspoon freshly ground pepper, divided
- ¼ teaspoon salt, divided
- ⅓ cup 1% milk
- ½ cup plain dry breadcrumbs
- portobello mushroom caps, 3-4 inches in diameter
- 3 cloves garlic, minced
- 1 pound spinach, tough stems removed
- 1 15-ounce can white beans, rinsed
- ¾ cup vegetable broth
- ½ cup grated Manchego, Gruyere or Parmesan cheese

Directions

1. Heat 1 tablespoon oil in a medium nonstick skillet over medium heat. Add onion and cook, stirring occasionally, until brown, 8 to 10 minutes. Reduce heat to very low, season with 1/4 teaspoon pepper and 1/8 teaspoon salt. Continue cooking, stirring occasionally, until caramelized, about 15 minutes Transfer to a bowl and keep warm.

2. Meanwhile, place milk in a small bowl and place breadcrumbs on a large plate. Dip each mushroom cap in milk, then dredge in the breadcrumbs.

3. Heat 1 tablespoon oil in a large nonstick skillet over medium heat. Add mushrooms, gill-side down. Place a heavy, heatproof plate or pie pan on top of the mushrooms and cook until golden brown, pressing down on the plate periodically to flatten them, about 6 minutes. Carefully remove the plate using an oven mitt or tongs, add 1 tablespoon oil to the pan and turn the mushrooms over. Replace the plate and cook, pressing the plate once or twice, until the mushrooms are golden brown and cooked through, 5

to 6 minutes more. Remove from heat; cover to keep warm.

4. Heat the remaining 1 tablespoon oil in a Dutch oven over medium-high heat. Add garlic and cook until fragrant, 20 to 30 seconds. Add spinach and cook, stirring, until just wilted, about 2 minutes. Stir in beans, broth and the remaining 1/4 teaspoon pepper and 1/8 teaspoon salt. Cook, stirring occasionally, until heated through, 1 to 2 minutes.

5. Cut each mushroom into thin slices and serve over the spinach. Top with the reserved onions and cheese.

27. Artichoke & Red Pepper Frittata

Total Time: 35 mins

Servings: 2

Ingredients

- 2 teaspoons extra-virgin olive oil, divided
- 1 medium red bell pepper, diced
- 2 cloves garlic, minced
- ¼ teaspoon crushed red pepper
- 4 large eggs
- 1 14-ounce can artichoke hearts, rinsed and coarsely chopped
- ¼ cup freshly grated Parmesan cheese
- 1 teaspoon dried oregano
- ¼ teaspoon salt, or to taste
- Freshly ground pepper, to taste

Directions

1 Heat 1 teaspoon oil in a 10-inch nonstick skillet over medium heat. Add bell pepper and cook until tender, about 2 minutes. Add garlic and crushed red pepper;

cook, stirring, for 30 seconds. Transfer to a plate. Wipe out the pan.

2   Whisk eggs in a medium bowl. Stir in artichoke hearts, Parmesan, oregano, salt, pepper and the bell pepper mixture.

3   Set a rack about 4 inches from the heat source; preheat the broiler.

4   Brush the pan with the remaining 1 teaspoon oil; heat over medium heat. Pour in the egg mixture and tilt to distribute evenly. Reduce the heat to medium-low and cook until the bottom is light golden, lifting the edges to allow uncooked egg to flow underneath, 3 to 4 minutes. Place the pan under the broiler and cook until the top is set, 1 1/2 to 2 1/2 minutes. Slide the frittata onto a platter and cut into wedges.

28. Roasted Pepper-&-Cheese Stuffed Chicken

Total Time: 40 mins

Servings: 4

Ingredients

- ⅓ cup chopped jarred roasted red peppers, rinsed
- ¼ cup shredded provolone cheese
- 2 boneless, skinless chicken breasts (about 1 1/4 pounds), trimmed
- ¾ teaspoon ground pepper, divided
- ½ teaspoon salt
- ½ teaspoon dried oregano
- 2 tablespoons extra-virgin olive oil, divided
- ounces whole-wheat orzo
-]¼ cup chopped Kalamata olives
- cups broccoli florets
- 2 tablespoons unsalted butter
- 4 lemon wedges, for serving

Directions

1   Preheat oven to 425 degrees F. Coat an 8-inch square baking dish with cooking spray.

2   Combine roasted peppers and provolone in a small bowl. Cut a horizontal slit along the thin, long edge of each chicken breast, nearly through to the opposite side. Season the chicken with 1/2 teaspoon pepper, salt and oregano. Fill each chicken breast "pocket" with half of the cheese mixture, and press the edges together to seal. Place the chicken in the prepared baking dish and drizzle with 1 tablespoon oil.

3   Bake the chicken until an instant-read thermometer inserted into the thickest part registers 165 degrees F, 20 to 25 minutes.

4   Meanwhile, cook orzo according to package directions. Drain; transfer to a bowl and toss with olives, the remaining 2 teaspoons oil and 1/4 teaspoon pepper.

5   Steam broccoli over 1 inch of boiling water in a pot fit with a steamer basket until just tender, 4 to 5 minutes. Transfer to a bowl and toss with butter.

6 Cut each chicken breast in half and serve with the orzo, the broccoli and lemon wedges, if desired.

29. Chickpea & Bulgur Stuffed Grape Leaves

Total Time: 2 hrs

Servings: 55

Ingredients

- 1 15- to 16-ounce jar grape leaves,drained
- Zest of 1 lemon
- ½ cup lemon juice, divided
- cloves garlic, peeled and halved
- 3 tablespoons tahini
- 2 tablespoons extra-virgin olive oil
- 1 tablespoon sumac
- 1 teaspoon freshly ground pepper
- ¾ teaspoon salt
- 1 19-ounce can chickpeas, rinsed
- ¾ cup bulgur
- ½ cup finely chopped fresh parsley
- scallions, trimmed and finely chopped
- Lemon wedges for serving
- Plain yogurt for serving

Directions

1   Put a large saucepan of water on to boil. Remove
    grape leaves from the jar and unroll. Separate into
    two piles--one of whole leaves and one with any torn
    leaves or pieces of leaves. The whole leaves will be
    used for rolling. Set aside the others for Step 5.

2   Cook the whole grape leaves in the boiling water for
    5 minutes; transfer with tongs to a colander to drain.

3   To prepare filling: Process lemon zest and 1/4 cup
    juice, garlic, tahini, oil, sumac (if using), pepper and
    salt in a food processor until smooth. Scrape into a
    large bowl. Pulse chickpeas in the food processor
    until coarsely chopped. Add to the lemon mixture
    along with bulgur, parsley and scallions; mix until
    well combined.

4   To assemble grape leaves: Lay a clean kitchen towel
    on a work surface. Place 4 to 6 whole grape leaves at
    a time on the towel with the stem-side up and stem
    end pointing toward you. Pinch or trim off any long
    or tough stems. Depending on the size of the leaf,
    shape 2 teaspoons to 1 tablespoon of the filling into a
    1 1/2- to 2-inch log and place it on the leaf,

perpendicular to the stem end. Roll the end of the leaf over the filling, tuck in the sides and roll tightly into a cigar shape. Repeat with the remaining grape leaves and filling. (You may have filling or grape leaves left over.)

5   Place the torn or very small leftover grape leaves in a large saucepan, covering the bottom completely; this will prevent the stuffed leaves from sticking as they cook. (No leftover leaves? See Tip.) Place about half of the stuffed grape leaves in one tight layer in the pan and drizzle with 2 tablespoons lemon juice. Make a second layer of grape leaves on top of the first and drizzle with the remaining 2 tablespoons lemon juice.

6   Place the largest heatproof plate you have that will fit in the pot on top of the grape leaves. Place a small-to-medium heatproof bowl on top of the plate and fill it three-quarters full with water (this will act as a weight to keep the grape leaves submerged). Add water to the pan until it reaches the rim of the plate.

7   Timing: Bring to a boil, then reduce heat to a simmer. Cook until the bulgur is tender, adding water as necessary to keep the grape leaves

submerged, about 30 minutes. (To check if the bulgur is done, carefully remove the bowl and plate, take out one stuffed grape leaf using a slotted spoon and cut it open.)

8   Carefully remove the bowl and plate, then transfer the grape leaves from the water using a slotted spoon. Serve warm with lemon wedges and yogurt for dipping, if desired.

30. Eggplant & Mozzarella Stick Roll-Ups

Total Time: 35 mins

Servings: 4

Ingredients

- frozen mozzarella sticks
- 1 medium eggplant (about 1 pound)
- ½ teaspoon kosher salt plus 1/8 teaspoon, divided
- 1 clove garlic, finely chopped
- 1 cup finely diced tomatoes
- ¼ cup finely chopped fresh basil, plus more for garnish
- ½ teaspoon ground pepper, divided
- 2 large eggs
- 2 tablespoons extra-virgin olive oil, divided

Directions

1   Preheat oven according to directions on mozzarella stick package.

2   Trim eggplant. Cut off the sides to make it somewhat rectangular and even, then cut lengthwise into eight

1/4-inch-thick slices. Place the slices on another baking sheet. Sprinkle with 1/4 teaspoon salt. Let stand for 10 minutes.

3 Mash garlic and 1/8 teaspoon salt with a fork. Transfer to a bowl and mix with tomatoes, basil and 1/4 teaspoon pepper. Set aside.

4 Bake mozzarella sticks according to package directions.

5 Meanwhile, blot the eggplant slices with paper towels. Sprinkle with the remaining 1/4 teaspoon each salt and pepper. Line another baking sheet with paper towels.

6 Lightly beat eggs in a shallow dish. Heat 1 tablespoon oil in a large nonstick skillet over medium-high heat. Dip 2 eggplant slices in the egg, letting excess drip off. Cook the eggplant until brown on both sides, 2 to 4 minutes total. Transfer to the paper-towel lined baking sheet. Repeat with 2 more eggplant slices. Add the remaining 1 tablespoon oil. Cook the remaining eggplant in 2 batches, adjusting heat as necessary.

7 Remove the paper towels from under the eggplant. Roll up a hot mozzarella stick in each eggplant slice.

Bake the roll-ups until hot, about 5 minutes. Serve with the reserved tomato sauce, garnished with basil, if desired.

www.ingramcontent.com/pod-product-compliance
Lightning Source LLC
Chambersburg PA
CBHW070958250726
48663CB00002B/280